your child's teeth

how to keep your child's teeth and gums healthy

Jane Kemp and Clare Walters

Consultant in Paediatric Dentistry: Kate Barnard

hamlyn

contents

First published in Great Britain
in 2003 by Hamlyn, a division
of Octopus Publishing Group Ltd
2–4 Heron Quays, London E14 4JP

Copyright © Octopus Publishing
Group Ltd 2003

ISBN 0 600 60665 1

A CIP catalogue record for this book is
available from the British Library

Printed and bound in China

10 9 8 7 6 5 4 3 2 1

Safety Note: While the advice and
information in this book is believed to
be accurate, neither the author nor
publisher can accept any legal
responsibility for any injury or illness
sustained while following the advice
within it.

INTRODUCTION   6

1 YOUR PREGNANCY   8
- Your growing baby   10
- What can affect your baby's teeth?   12
- Taking care of yourself   14
- Safety precautions   18

2 UNDERSTANDING YOUR CHILD'S TEETH   20
- How your child's teeth emerge   22
- The tooth and its supporting tissues   25
- The jaw and gums   27
- Why milk teeth matter   28
- How feeding affects tooth development   30

3 TEETHING   34
- Starting to teethe   36
- Teething or illness?   38
- Soothing your baby   40
- Relieving teething pain   42

4 HOW TO KEEP TEETH CLEAN   44
- Starting to clean   46
- Your growing child   47
- Get brushing right   50
- Choosing a toothbrush   52

5 PREVENTING DECAY   **54**
  • Tooth decay explained   56
  • Periodontal disease   58
  • How to prevent decay   59

6 VISITING THE DENTIST   **66**
  • Finding the right dentist   68
  • The first visit   70
  • First fillings   72
  • Further visits and procedures   74

7 OTHER PROBLEMS WITH TEETH   **76**
  • Medical problems   78
  • Other teeth troubles   80
  • Losing or breaking a tooth   84
  • Childhood habits   86
  • When will they wobble?   88
  • Problem-solving: questions and answers   89

TOP 10 TIPS   92
INDEX   94
ACKNOWLEDGEMENTS   96

Introduction

This book will help you to care for your child's teeth and gums, from birth through to a full set of milk teeth – and beyond, to the first hint of a wobble!

There are few things as exciting as seeing that first milk tooth beginning to appear in your baby's mouth. From the start, you will need to take great care over your child's teeth and gums, as you will be establishing healthy hygiene routines right from the word go.

But long before you see that first tiny tooth, your baby's teeth will have been forming, since you were around 4 months pregnant, so it is very important to care for yourself during pregnancy. In Chapter 1 you will find lots of helpful advice for eating a balanced diet, plus other tips on caring for yourself and your growing baby during this special time.

Of course, your baby is unlikely to be born with teeth, but it won't be long before you see that first pearly-white glimmer. In Chapter 2 we tell you when to expect each new tooth to appear and how to keep your baby's whole mouth healthy. Then, when those teeth do start to come through, Chapter 3 provides plenty of advice for soothing the discomfort that teething may cause your baby.

One of the key things you will want to know is how to keep your baby's teeth clean. Chapter 4 explains how to choose the right toothbrush and toothpaste, as well as how to perfect the brushing technique. There are also tips for getting reluctant toddlers to brush! Then Chapter 5 looks at the best ways to protect your child's teeth from decay, including being careful about what they eat and drink and ensuring vital fluoride protection.

Getting to know your dentist is an essential part of long-term tooth care, so in Chapter 6 we help you

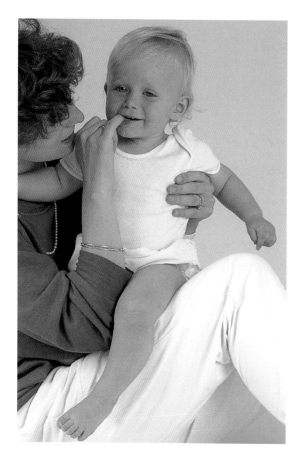

Left Your baby's first tooth is most likely to appear at any time from six months onwards.

to find the right dentist, explain how to make the first visit go smoothly, tell you what the dentist will do, and provide advice on how to cope if your child does need a filling.

Despite the best care, you may encounter problems with your child's teeth, so in the final chapter we look at other some of the potential difficulties, and also provide tips on breaking habits like thumb-sucking that can affect your child's teeth and gums.

We hope you enjoy this book and find it helpful as you look after your child's teeth.

your
pregnancy

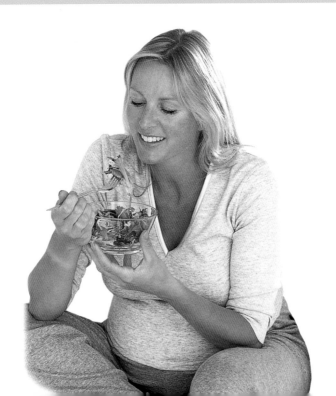

1

- Your growing baby

- What can affect your baby's teeth?

- Taking care of yourself

- Safety precautions

Your growing baby

A balanced diet, regular gentle exercise and plenty of rest are the basic ingredients of a healthy pregnancy. Understanding how your baby grows, and how early on his teeth are forming, will help you to realize that if you stay fit and well during pregnancy you are giving your baby the best possible start.

How your baby's teeth develop in the womb

1 By the time your baby has been growing for 4 months his teeth are starting to form. Your baby absorbs calcium and phosphate from your blood stream which 'mineralize' into teeth. Vitamin D and growth hormones are also an essential part of the process.

2 Although milk teeth don't usually appear in your baby's mouth until around 6 months after birth, parts of all 20 of his milk teeth are formed before he is born. These milk teeth begin life as tooth buds, from which the crowns – the visible part of the tooth that you can see in the mouth – begin to form.

3 The teeth grow in the jaws in little sacs called 'follicles'.

4 When the crowns are complete, the roots of the teeth begin to develop. Root formation is finally completed sometime after the teeth come through (erupt) and are fully hardened. The enamel coating on the teeth is the hardest tissue in the body and is stronger than iron!

'At my first appointment after I discovered I was pregnant my doctor told me that I was entitled to free dental treatment. I hadn't realized this and it seemed a good opportunity to 'catch up', as I hadn't been to the dentist for several years. I was a bit nervous to begin with but it was fine – the dentist asked me lots of questions before examining me, and gave me plenty of advice about flossing (which I'd never done before). I'll definitely go back after the baby's born.'

Julie, 8 months pregnant

The sucking reflex

Antenatal scans often show babies sucking their thumbs or fingers. This is a natural way for your baby to practise the jaw and mouth movements he will need after birth.

After birth, the strong tongue and lip actions your baby uses during feeding stimulate the growth of his jaws. At this stage his first adult teeth are already beginning to form in his gums.

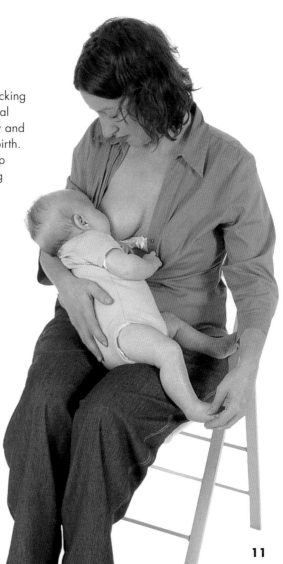

Right:
Breastfeeding gives your baby the best possible start, and helps to protect against infections.

What can affect your baby's teeth?

You do not need to do anything special to help your baby's teeth grow well, beyond looking after yourself and eating a balanced diet. However, there are some events that can have a direct effect on how her teeth develop.

Mercury alert

Most ordinary silver fillings contain tiny amounts of mercury, which is a poisonous metal. Although the amounts are so small that these fillings are still considered safe, mercury can cross the placenta, so you are advised to avoid any dental work involving amalgam while pregnant.

Infections

If you contract a viral or bacterial infection, the development of the tooth germ may be disturbed. To avoid infections in pregnancy as far as possible, see *Foods to avoid* on page 18.

Premature birth

There is now some evidence to suggest that premature birth and low birth weight may affect the development of those teeth which are developing during the perinatal period. A pre-term baby may be missing out on an extra build-up of minerals.

Drugs and X-rays

Medical and dental professionals are now well aware of the risks posed to the unborn baby's teeth by giving a pregnant women antibiotics containing tetracycline. These can cause discoloration of whichever of the baby's teeth are developing at the time, but this will become evident only once the teeth erupt. This means that it is very important to inform any health professional as soon as you know you are pregnant.

If you're already on long-term medication for a specific medical condition, such as epilepsy or a thyroid problem, it's best to talk to your GP or hospital staff to let them know that you're planning to become pregnant. This will enable them to assess the most appropriate treatment for you in pregnancy.

X-rays may also affect an unborn baby's development, so again you must let health staff know you are pregnant – or even that you might be pregnant – before undergoing any X-ray procedure, such as a dental X-ray or a hospital investigation if, for example, you have an suspected fracture.

Newborn (natal) teeth

Occasionally babies are born with one or two teeth already visible. These are not extra teeth but simply milk teeth that are growing close to the surface of the gum.

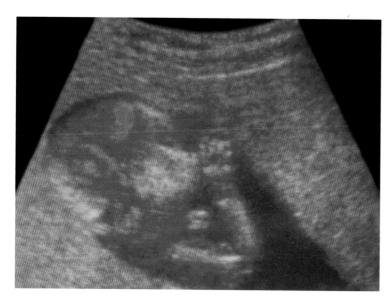

Left: Even in the womb, your baby's teeth are already forming in the jaw.

Taking care of yourself

To give your baby the best chance of growing well, and thereby developing healthy teeth, there are a number of steps you can take during your pregnancy.

- **Take folic acid.** A daily 400mcg supplement is recommended both before you become pregnant and for the first 12 weeks of your pregnancy. This helps to reduce the risk of spinal defects such as spina bifida.
- **Stop smoking.** Your baby's development and growth are adversely affected by smoking, so stop smoking if you can, or cut down as much as possible. Your doctor can offer advice and guidance to help you quit.
- **Cut right down on alcohol.** Stick to a maximum of one or two units a week: a unit is equivalent to one glass of wine or 250ml (½ pint) of beer.
- **Exercise sensibly.** You can continue to enjoy moderate exercise like swimming or walking when you are pregnant, but don't take up a new or vigorous exercise programme without seeking advice from your doctor.
- **Cut down on caffeine.** Avoid drinking tea, coffee or cola as much as possible. Higher caffeine levels have been linked with a risk of miscarriage.

A healthy diet

Your baby needs to receive a combination of calcium, phosphorus and other minerals and vitamins in order to develop strong teeth. As your baby's teeth are already forming from as early as 4 months into your pregnancy, making sure your diet contains essential nutrients can affect their development right from the start.

Extra calories

For the first 6 months of pregnancy your body is super-efficient at absorbing the nutrients you need from your usual diet. During the last 3 months you will need an extra 200 calories per day. Overall, the rule in pregnancy is to eat when you are hungry, and eat healthily.

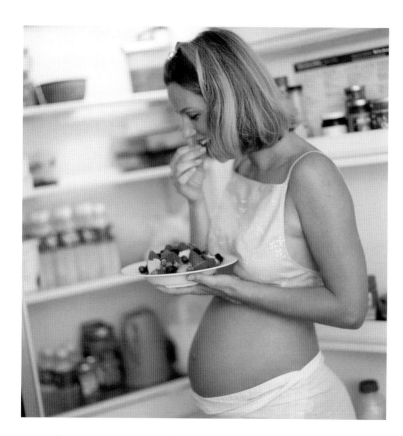

Left: *Taking care over your diet in pregnancy will give you more energy, and promote your baby's healthy growth.*

Foods containing fat and sugar

Essential fatty acids are contained in many foods, such as meat, oily fish and dairy foods. However, many foods contain high levels of saturated fat, and too much of this can be bad for you.

If you eat a good selection from the four food groups (see pages 16–17), you will get the fatty acids you need. Cakes, biscuits and processed foods, such as pork pies, contain high levels of saturated fat, so keep these to a minimum. Similarly, watch how many sugary foods you are eating.

To reduce your fat intake, remove the skin from a chicken portion, cut off visible fat from meat, and use low-fat or semi-skimmed dairy products.

Free treatment

Check with your doctor or dentist to see if you are eligible to receive free dental treatment during pregnancy and following the birth of your baby.

15

Food group	How much?
Bread, cereals (including breakfast cereals), potatoes, pasta, rice and noodles	4–6 servings per day. A serving is equivalent to either a bowl of cereal, a couple of potatoes, a portion of pasta or rice, or two slices of bread. Include these foods in every meal, to make up around one-third of your daily food intake.
Fruit and vegetables	5 servings per day. Try to include dark green and orange-coloured vegetables and/or fruit. Cook vegetables for the minimum length of time and eat as soon as possible after cooking. Eat some fresh fruit and raw vegetables every day.
Meat, fish, eggs, nuts, pulses (baked beans, lentils, chickpeas, red kidney beans, etc.)	2–3 servings per day.
Milk and dairy foods (cheese, yogurt, butter, etc.)	2–3 servings per day. A serving is equivalent to 250ml (½ pint) of fresh milk, a small pot of yogurt or 40g (1½oz) of hard cheese.

Why it is important	Tips
Source of carbohydrates, protein and B vitamins. Low in fat, filling and relatively inexpensive. Valuable source of dietary fibre.	Choose wholegrain varieties where possible, as these contain more dietary fibre.
Contain a range of vitamins (including vitamin C, carotene and B group vitamins) and other nutrients, as well as the dietary fibre needed in pregnancy.	Do not store for too long, as vitamins are lost relatively quickly. Fruit and vegetable juices provide the vitamins and minerals, but lack dietary fibre.
Excellent source of protein as well as minerals and vitamins.	Choose lean meat and trim off fat. Grill or bake rather than fry. If you are vegetarian, make sure you replace meat and fish with other good sources of protein.
Especially high in calcium but also contain vitamins and protein.	Dairy alternatives include enriched soya milk and soya products, tofu, beans and sesame seeds, green vegetables (especially spinach), dried fruit, fish eaten with bones (e.g. tinned sardines). Low-fat versions provide just as much calcium as the full-fat equivalent, so choose these if you are concerned about weight gain.

Safety precautions

You can protect yourself and your baby from food poisoning and infections, some of which may affect the development of his teeth (see page 12), by following the simple precautions outlined on these pages. Although the list of foods below may appear long, remember you'll only have to steer clear of them during pregnancy, and once your baby is born, you'll be able to enjoy all your favourite treats again.

Ouch!

Hormonal changes in pregnancy make your gums more prone to inflammation and you may notice that they bleed when you brush your teeth. This is normal, but take extra care with brushing and flossing.

Foods to avoid

- **Liver and liver products**, including cod liver oil and liver pâté. These are high in vitamin A (retinol), which can damage the developing baby early in your pregnancy, including an increased risk of cleft lip and palate.
- **Soft, mould-ripened cheeses** such as Camembert, Brie and blue-veined cheese. These may contain listeria, which can cause a disease that may affect your baby.
- **All types of fresh pâté**, including all meat and vegetable varieties. These can also contain listeria.
- **Raw and lightly cooked eggs**. These may contain salmonella, which can cause sickness and diarrhoea, so are best avoided.
- **Unpasteurized milk**. This may harbour dangerous 'bugs', including tuberculosis (TB).
- **Raw shellfish**. These can contain harmful bacteria and viruses.

Take special care

You will need to be extra-cautious about food hygiene and preparation during your pregnancy. Be aware of these key 'musts' in the kitchen:

Reheat cooked, chilled ready-meals to piping hot to destroy any bacteria.

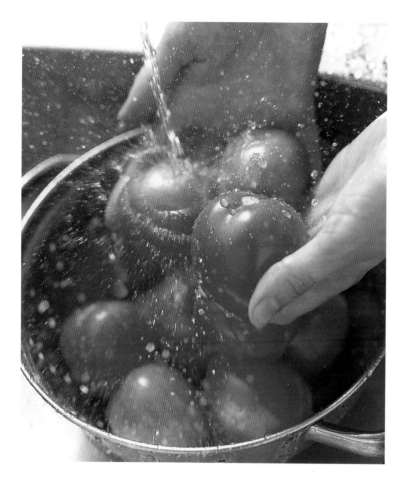

Left: Protect yourself from potential infection by taking special care to wash fresh fruit and vegetables thoroughly in cold running water.

2 Store raw poultry and meat at the lowest level in your refrigerator to avoid contamination of other foods, and always wash your hands after handling, as they may contain bacteria, including salmonella.

3 Wash vegetables (especially salads) thoroughly to remove debris which could contain micro-organisms such as toxoplasmosis – a disease often transmitted through cat faeces – that can affect your unborn baby.

Allergy alert

If you or the baby's father have a family history of allergies, avoid eating peanuts or peanut products while you are pregnant or breastfeeding.

understanding your child's teeth

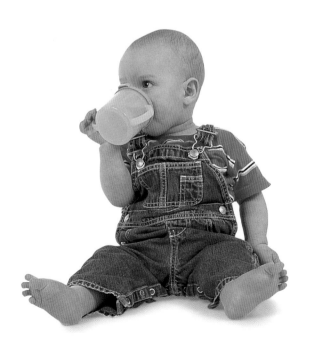

2

- How your child's teeth emerge

- The tooth and its supporting tissues

- The jaw and gums

- Why milk teeth matter

- How feeding affects tooth development

How your child's teeth emerge

It's a really exciting day when you notice a hint of white emerging from your baby's gum – the first tiny tooth coming through, leading the way for the full set of 20 baby or 'milk' teeth that will last for at least 5 years, and some for up to 12 years.

Your baby's milk teeth are essential to provide the right foundation for the later permanent teeth.

1 For most children (though not all), the first milk tooth will appear at around 6 months of age. It may appear suddenly, but more usually it is preceded by a bump beneath the gum before it erupts.

2 The two front teeth at the bottom usually come through first, quickly followed by the two front teeth at the top. These four teeth are known as the central incisors and are used for biting. Once these initial teeth have appeared, you can expect to see the teeth on either side of the central incisors coming through next, often two at a time. These are called the lateral incisors. Your baby will now have eight teeth.

3 The next teeth you can expect to see are the four back teeth – the first molars. Two appear in the lower jaw, followed by two in the upper jaw. These are the teeth your baby will use for chewing, which is why they have flat grinding surfaces.

4 Next, the longer, pointed teeth – the canines – emerge in both jaws.

5 Lastly, the second set of four molars erupt at the very back of your child's mouth, giving her the grand total of 20 milk teeth!

'My baby didn't have a tooth at all on her first birthday, and I was beginning to wonder whether she'd ever get one! But within a month the first one appeared at the front of her top jaw, and several others quickly followed. She learned to walk in the same week that she got her first tooth, so we had a double celebration.'

Kerry, mother of Ruby (18 months)

Which teeth when?

The diagram on the next page shows the order in which your baby's teeth will emerge. It also gives the approximate age at which you might expect to see them come through. However, it's worth remembering that teeth may appear 6 months earlier or later than these ages and still be within the normal range.

Milk teeth have to last a long time. From the first one emerging when your baby is around 6 months old, it will be a wait of some 6 years before the first one is lost, to be replaced by a permanent tooth. Your child is likely to lose teeth in roughly the same order that they arrived, but this happens gradually over a period of around 6 years, between the ages of 6 and 12. The chart on the next page shows when they might fall out.

Because a permanent tooth doesn't always arrive straight after your child has lost a milk tooth, you'll see the characteristic gappy grin. Again, the chart on the next page gives an idea of when to expect those 32 permanent teeth to erupt: 16 on the upper jaw and 16 on the lower jaw.

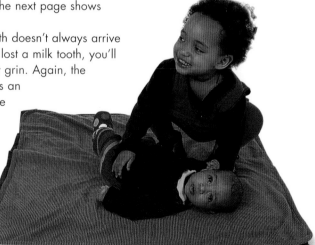

Below: Those first teeth will take your baby right through her toddler years and beyond.

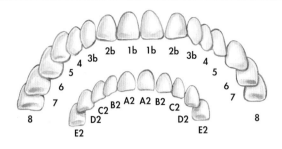

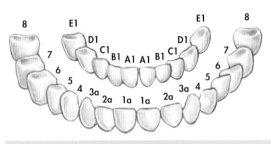

Permanent teeth

Tooth	Growing
1a Central incisors, lower	6–7 years
1b Central incisors, upper	7–8 years
2a Lateral incisors, lower	6–7 years
2b Lateral incisors, upper	8–9 years
4 First pre-molars	10–12 years
5 Second pre-molars	10–12 years
3a Canines, lower	10 years
3b Canines, upper	11–12 years
6 First molars	6 years
7 Second molars	11–13 years
8 Third molars	17 years+

Milk teeth

Tooth	Growing	Losing
A1 Central incisors, lower	6 months	6–7 years
A2 Central incisors, upper	7½ months	7–8 years
B1 Lateral incisors, lower	7 months	6–7 years
B2 Lateral incisors, upper	9 months	8–9 years
D1 First molars, lower	12 months	9–10 years
D2 First molars, upper	14 months	9–10 years
C1 Canines, lower	16 months	10 years
C2 Canines, upper	18 months	11 years
E1 Second molars, lower	20 months	10–11 years
E2 Second molars, upper	2 years	10–11 years

The tooth and its supporting tissues

As you can see from the diagram on page 26, a tooth is made up of a number of different materials. It is divided into three basic parts: the crown is the part of the tooth that you can see; the neck is the area where the tooth disappears into the gum; and the root is hidden within the bone of the jaw. The tooth is made up of enamel, dentine, pulp and cementum, and is held in the jaw by supporting fibres known as the periodontal ligament.

The enamel

The crown of the tooth is protected by a layer of enamel, which is thicker at the top and becomes thinner towards the neck, where the tooth meets the jaw. Its main job is to protect the other tissues inside the teeth, and to absorb the considerable impact of biting and chewing.

Enamel is an amazingly hard substance, made up of minerals in crystalline form, that is affected very little by changes in temperature.

In young children, the enamel is especially thin at the bottom of the tiny grooves and fissures that you'll see on the biting surfaces of the molars. Also, enamel is not distributed evenly over the tooth, and tiny pits and irregularities can become traps for food and plaque. These areas are the ones most likely to become decayed, which is why it is so important not to overlook cleaning every surface of every tooth.

The dentine

Directly under the enamel is the dentine, which extends right down into the root of the tooth. The dentine forms the main part of the tooth and is made from a similar substance to the enamel.

White – or not quite?

The colour of your teeth is linked with the thickness of the enamel covering. If the enamel layer is thin, the yellow-coloured dentine shows through more clearly, giving the teeth a yellowish tint. White teeth aren't necessarily stronger than yellowish teeth, nor are they less likely to be affected by decay.

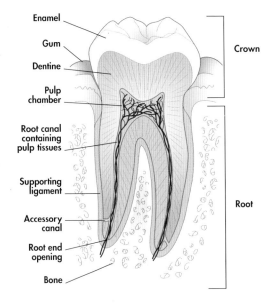

Enamel

Gum

Dentine

Pulp
chamber

Root canal
containing
pulp tissues

Supporting
ligament

Accessory
canal

Root end
opening

Bone

Crown

Root

However, it is more yellow and less hard than the enamel.

The dentine is very sensitive and is highly responsive to changes in temperature, which is why it hurts when you have a cavity or gum recession where the dentine is exposed.

The pulp

Packed with nerves and blood vessels, the pulp forms the central part of the tooth. It is extremely sensitive, and its nerve cells when stimulated transmit pain signals to the brain.

The cementum

As its name suggests, this bone-like substance is connected to the supporting jawbone by fibres known as the periodontal ligament. It covers and protects the root of the tooth, in much the same way as enamel does the crown, although cementum is not as hard as enamel. Cementum continues to form throughout life, but may be exposed by receding gums and can be worn down by over-vigorous brushing.

Supporting fibres

These fibres may be destroyed or damaged by inflammation or infection, which may cause the tooth to become loose or painful.

The jaw and gums

The jaws form the framework of the mouth and contain the teeth.

The gums cover and protect the jawbones.

The jaw

The upper jaw is called the maxilla and is fixed to the base of the skull. The lower jaw is called the mandible and can move in a variety of directions to allow for biting, chewing and speaking. The upper and lower jaws grow with your child to allow room for the second set of teeth to emerge as she approaches puberty. Ideally, the two jaws should relate efficiently so that the upper and lower teeth act together in biting and chewing.

The gums

The gums, also known as gingivae, are made of soft tissues – both 'attached' and 'non-attached' – which cover the bone. Healthy gums are a pale pink colour and are attached to the teeth and bound to the jawbone. Bacteria in plaque can cause the gums to become red and swollen, forming 'pockets' that can quickly become plaque traps.

One of the most obvious signs of inflammation is bleeding gums, which can discourage brushing, but gentle brushing at least twice a day is even more important now. Your 'tooth' brush should actually be a 'gum' brush as well and should be small-headed with soft nylon 'bristles'.

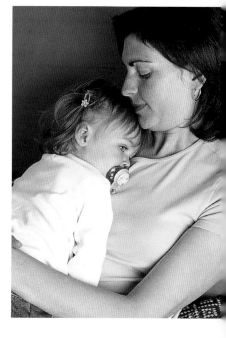

Above: *If your child uses a dummy, try to restrict it to sleep and nap times, and remove it once she's asleep.*

Why milk teeth matter

Your baby's milk teeth are very important – and not just because they look nice. Taking care of them right from the start will give your child the best possible chance of having a healthy mouth and strong teeth right into adulthood.

Here are the key reasons why these first teeth matter so much for your child.

Maintaining spacing

The milk teeth maintain space into which the permanent teeth may grow. If one is missing, it may be necessary for your child to wear a brace or 'space maintainer' to hold space for the adult tooth. Teeth 'drift' when space becomes available due to the untimely loss of teeth.

Below: Eating family meals together will encourage your child to enjoy mealtimes as sociable occasions.

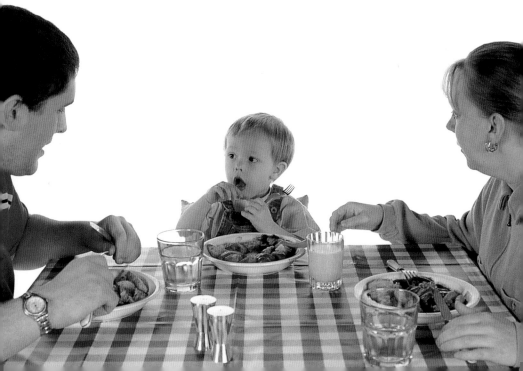

Growing and developing

Teeth influence the shape of your child's face. They are important cosmetically, too: a child who is self-conscious about his teeth will simply be unwilling to smile.

Eating well

As your baby moves on to solids, his teeth will become increasingly important as he develops the skills of biting, chewing and grinding. Teeth also play a role in normal speech development.

Protecting permanent teeth

Caring for milk teeth will help to give your child a healthy mouth for the permanent teeth. An infection of a milk tooth could cause damage to the permanent tooth that is developing in the jaw. An abscess on a milk tooth root could 'scar' the permanent tooth directly underneath before it has even emerged, by disturbing its development.

A long job

Some of the milk teeth are intended to be in your child's mouth for 10–12 years (see pages 22–24) so it is important that these teeth remain healthy throughout this time.

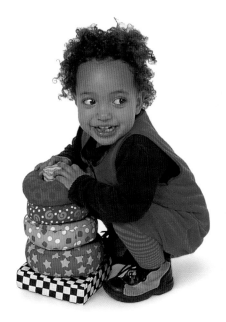

Above: Healthy teeth help to give your child a happy confident smile.

How feeding affects tooth development

The action your baby uses to feed, whether from a bottle or the breast, helps her jaw to grow and also develops the muscles in the cheeks that she will need for chewing food and talking. It is interesting to compare the different techniques your baby uses to feed from a breast and a bottle.

Breastfeeding

Breastfeeding is best for your baby. Human breast milk is exactly the right food for her, and helps her immune system.

Here is the best way to position your baby at the breast:

1 Make sure she is on her side with her mouth directly opposite your nipple. Her head should be in line with her body so that she is close to you.

2 Brush her cheek with your nipple to encourage her to open her mouth wide, then draw her on to your breast. Her tongue should rest on her bottom lip so that it is underneath the nipple as she feeds.

Constant feeding

Remember that breast milk is sweet and will cause decay in your baby's newly erupting teeth if she is constantly feeding.

3 If it feels uncomfortable, or her mouth isn't open wide enough and she simply seems to be 'nibbling' rather than feeding, slip your little finger into the corner of her mouth to break the suction and try latching her on again. Her mouth should cover all the nipple and a good part of the areola too (the dark area around the nipple). As she feeds, you will notice her jaw moving or her ears wiggling as the jaw muscles work to draw the milk from your breast.

If your baby bites your breast while feeding, say 'no' in a calm, firm voice and remove her from the breast, using a finger in the corner of her mouth to break the suction. Hard gums can be just as painful as teeth, so if your baby is biting too hard, use the same technique, but make sure you are offering enough teething toys or firm finger foods to help her explore this side of her development.

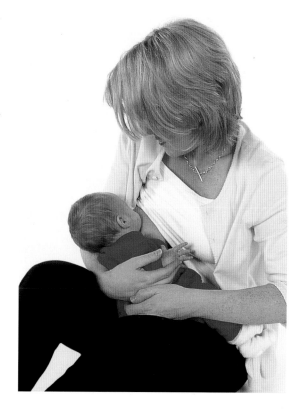

Above: *Breastfeeding is best for your baby and encourages her to use her lips and jaw as she sucks.*

Time for a cup

Switch to a feeding cup by the time your baby is a year old, as prolonged sucking of a nipple, teat, dummy or thumb may all lead to a prominent upper jaw and protruding teeth.

Bottlefeeding

If you are bottlefeeding, it's important to have your baby in a slightly more upright position so that the milk is swallowed easily and doesn't spend too much time swishing around in his mouth. You may want to choose an orthodontic teat that is designed to match a human nipple shape and encourages your baby to work his jaws in the same way that he would when breastfeeding.

Never leave your baby with a bottle of milk as a way of settling him. Not only is there a danger of choking, but leaving milk in his mouth for long periods will quickly result in tooth decay, sometimes known as 'bottle caries'.

What is the difference?

Breastfeeding	Bottlefeeding
Mouth open wide	Mouth only slightly open
Whole jaw involved in sucking	Jaw quite still
Lips fairly still	Lips do most of the work
Tongue moves to release milk from the breast	Tongue relatively still
Requires effort	Relatively easy for the baby

Super saliva

Saliva isn't just for keeping the mouth moist:

- Saliva is rich in minerals – calcium, phosphate and fluoride – which can help to rebuild tooth enamel in the early stages of decay.

- The fluoride also helps to protect the teeth from decay.

- Saliva has a cleansing effect after eating, and its lubricating effect makes chewing and swallowing easier.

- Saliva has a buffering function which neutralizes acids formed in the mouth.

- The amount of saliva in your mouth drops when you are thirsty, encouraging you to drink.

- One of its most important functions is to begin the process of digestion. Saliva contains enzymes that start to break down the food before it has even been swallowed.

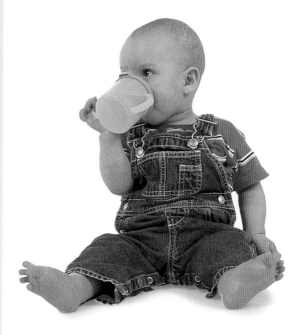

Above: *It's important to introduce a beaker as soon as possible – most babies can hold a beaker from 6 months old.*

teething

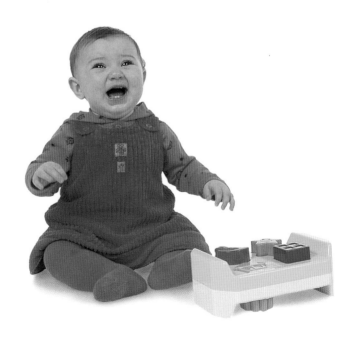

3

- Starting to teethe

- Teething or illness?

- Soothing your baby

- Relieving teething pain

Starting to teethe

Some people will tell you that teething is a normal physiological process with no adverse side effects. However, many parents will vouch for the distress it can cause.

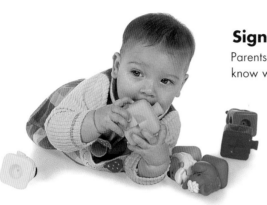

Signs of teething

Parents of first babies often ask how they will know when their baby is teething. If your baby is the right age and you spot any of the signs below, it's a fairly safe bet that a tooth is on its way.

Above: *You may notice your baby chewing or biting vigorously on her toys as a new tooth erupts.*

Munch, munch!

You can encourage your baby's biting and chewing skills even before the first tooth comes through by offering her tempting finger foods and toys with chewy bits and interesting textures to mouth. Check the age range of any toys carefully, and keep them clean with hot, soapy water between use.

- **In pain.** Your baby may show signs that she is in pain and is feeling uncomfortable.
- **Being irritable.** The discomfort of teething can make your baby grumpy and grizzly, and she may seem more clingy than usual a day or two before the tooth comes through.
- **A red cheek.** You may notice a reddish patch on your baby's cheek.
- **Dribbling.** The excess saliva that is produced during teething will make your baby drool.
- **Gnawing, chewing or biting.** Your baby may do this on anything that comes near her mouth.
- **Swollen gums.** Check inside her mouth to see if there is a slightly inflamed or puffy area on her gum.

- **Waking up.** Your baby may wake at night and seem fretful, even if she had been sleeping through regularly.
- **A raised temperature.** Teething is now recognized as causing a slightly raised temperature, so your baby may feel a little hotter than usual.
- **Sore bottom.** It's not clear why, but some parents notice that their babies seem more prone to nappy rash during a bout of teething, and may also have runny poo.

Want to see that new tooth?

If you want to see your baby's tooth before it emerges from the gum, press a clean finger firmly on the gum and quickly take it away to see the outline of the tooth below.

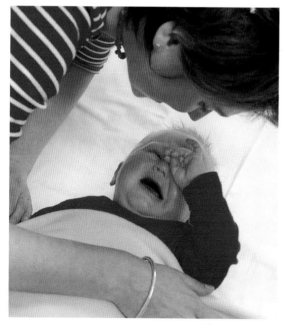

Left: Teething may make your baby feel uncomfortable but there's lots you can do to relieve his discomfort.

Teething or illness?

When your baby is hot and fretful, it can be easy to put his symptoms down to teething. But while it is true that teething may cause discomfort and irritability, it doesn't actually cause illness. So it is important to be able to recognize if your baby is unwell and to act promptly. If he is suffering from any of the symptoms below, be sure to take him to your doctor for a check-up:

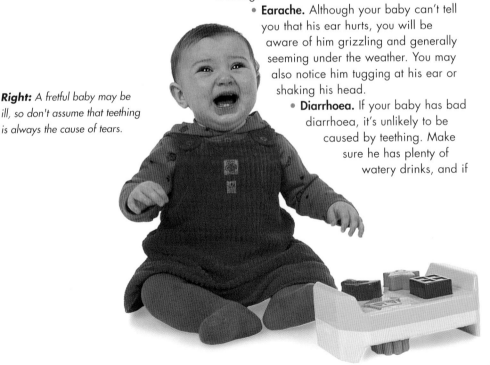

- **Prolonged crying.** This is your baby's principal way of telling you something is wrong. If he is inconsolable, he is probably feeling really unwell and you should not assume that this is due to teething.

- **Earache.** Although your baby can't tell you that his ear hurts, you will be aware of him grizzling and generally seeming under the weather. You may also notice him tugging at his ear or shaking his head.

- **Diarrhoea.** If your baby has bad diarrhoea, it's unlikely to be caused by teething. Make sure he has plenty of watery drinks, and if

Right: A fretful baby may be ill, so don't assume that teething is always the cause of tears.

he produces more than two runny faeces in a row take him to your doctor immediately.

- **Fever.** Teething can be associated with a slight rise in temperature, but if your baby has a fever of 38°C (100.4°F) or above this is much more likely to be caused by an infection, which could need treatment. If the fever persists for more than 24 hours, consult your doctor.
- **Refusing feeds.** Your baby may find feeding slightly uncomfortable when teething but he shouldn't refuse more than one feed, especially if you have taken steps to relieve any discomfort before starting the feed (see page 42).
- **Cough.** A cough is nearly always a sign of illness, although the excess saliva caused by dribbling from teething may make your baby cough and splutter a little. However, any breathing difficulty may have serious implications and you must consult your doctor.

Keep your baby comfortable

To help keep your baby comfortable:

- Give him a dose of infant paracetamol, checking the packaging for the correct dosage for your baby's age. Remember that aspirin-based products should never be given to a baby.
- Strip your baby down to a vest and nappy to help lower his temperature naturally.
- You may want to sponge him gently with warm (not cold) water, which will also help to reduce his temperature.
- If his temperature continues to rise, it is not caused by teething and you *must* consult your doctor.

Is it crooked?

It's perfectly natural for first teeth to look as if they are coming through in a slightly awkward fashion. They will continue to move and straighten out of their own accord. Also be prepared for them to be very sharp at first!

Let the dentist know

If your child has been ill during his first year, or if you were ill during pregnancy or experienced a difficult birth, let your dentist know about this when you visit. These events may have had an effect on the way the teeth mineralized as they formed, so they may need special attention.

Soothing your baby

An irritable baby can make everyone miserable. While some lucky babies sail through teething with scarcely a murmur, many suffer discomfort and need lots of love and comforting.

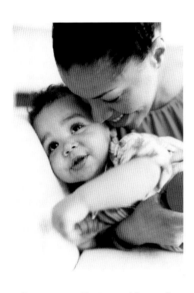

Above: Lots of loving cuddles and a gentle lullaby may be just what your baby needs to settle her.

Here are some simple ways to soothe a fretful baby which may also help get her to sleep:

- **Rocking.** Hold your baby close to you and rock her gently to and fro. She may like to be held lying in your arms or prefer to be upright against your shoulders. If your baby isn't too heavy, you may want to hold her in a baby carrier so that she feels really secure.
- **Singing.** The sound of your voice is always soothing for your baby, and if you sing soft songs or chat quietly to her she will want to listen, which in turn distracts her from feeling grumpy.
- **A mobile.** Something intriguing to look at may help your baby, so put a musical or light-themed mobile out of reach above her cot or pram.
- **Noise.** A gentle, droning background noise can actually soothe some babies. Sounds like the washing machine, vacuum cleaner or tumble dryer may appeal, so sit your baby in her bouncy chair nearby.
- **Distraction.** Let her watch you as you get on with household jobs, and keep chatting to her as you work. She'll also enjoy watching other children playing, so a visit to a mother-and-baby group may help.
- **Music.** Familiar music distracts as well as soothes, so put on a favourite tune or nursery rhyme tape.
- **Too cold?** Use a room thermometer to keep an eye on the temperature of your baby's room (ideally, around 18°C/64°F), and if it is too cold adjust her bedding accordingly.

- **Too hot?** Check that your baby isn't running a temperature. If she is, follow the tips in *Keep your baby comfortable* on page 39. Use a thermometer or simply slip your hand behind your baby's neck to judge whether or not she is too hot.
- **Sleeping alone.** If you can get your baby into the habit of settling herself, life will be a lot easier. To do this, lay your baby down to sleep when she is still awake, but drowsy. This may not work at first but will pay off in the long run, as it teaches your baby that she can fall asleep on her own. This in turn will help her get back to sleep quickly without crying if she wakes in the night due to discomfort from teething.
- **Getting out.** Any regular movement helps to settle a fretful baby. Wheel her out in her pram or go for a drive in the car to take her mind off her troubles.

Thirsty baby

Your baby is likely to drool a lot while teething and this means that she is losing a lot of extra fluids, so it's essential to keep offering plenty of extra breastfeeds or drinks of cooled, boiled water to prevent her becoming dehydrated.

Can a dummy help?

Sucking, biting or chewing on something can help soothe a teething baby. Suitable items can include a dummy, but try to limit a dummy to bed and nap times as prolonged use may result in a prominent upper jaw and protruding teeth. Once she's asleep, gently remove the dummy from her mouth.

- Never put a ribbon or other tie around your baby's neck to secure the dummy, as this could pose a real risk of strangulation – use a specially made dummy clip instead.

- Check dummies regularly for wear and tear, and throw them away as soon as there is any sign of damage.

- Sterilize dummies after each use, and store them in a special dummy case – never put a dummy back in your baby's mouth after it has fallen on the floor.

- Never sweeten the dummy before giving it to your baby as this will inevitably lead to tooth decay.

Relieving teething pain

It's always upsetting to hear your baby crying, but when you suspect that it might be teething pain that is causing his distress you'll be particularly anxious to do all you can to relieve the pain and stop the tears.

Here are some practical ways in which you may be able to help your baby:

- Buy two or three water-filled teething rings and keep them cool in the refrigerator (not the freezer, as this could cause ice 'burn'). Offer one to your baby if he seems to want something to gnaw on.
- Wash your hands well, then massage your baby's gums gently with your finger. You may even feel the bump in his gum where the tooth is about to emerge.
- Give him a quick breastfeed.

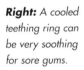

Right: A cooled teething ring can be very soothing for sore gums.

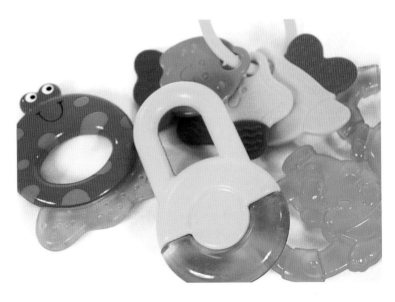

- Try rubbing a teething gel or liquid on to his gums, but don't do this more than 4–6 times a day. Always read the instructions on the packaging.
- Rub a partly thawed ice cube over your baby's gums. *Never leave him to suck the ice cube as he could choke.*
- Buy a baby 'finger toothbrush' and rub his gums gently with it. You can use this to keep the tooth clean once it is through.
- Offer crunchy finger foods for your baby to gnaw on. Try toast, lightly cooked carrot or apple slices, and always stay with your baby while he is eating to make sure he doesn't choke.
- If you are convinced that it is teething that is causing your baby discomfort, try giving him a dose of sugar-free infant paracetamol to see if it stops the pain.

'Both my boys found teething painful on occasions. If I felt they were really distressed I used a teething gel, and occasionally gave them some infant paracetamol.'

Caroline, mother of Spike (5) and Barney (3)

At the end of your tether?

If you are finding the crying and grizzling overwhelming, it won't do your baby any harm to be left in his cot for 5–10 minutes while you take a breather out of earshot. If you are finding life hard going, ask for help from friends, family or your partner – and don't forget that your health visitor is there to offer support. No one will criticize you for seeking help. Remember that however bad things get, you must never shake your baby, as this can cause him permanent damage.

how to keep teeth clean

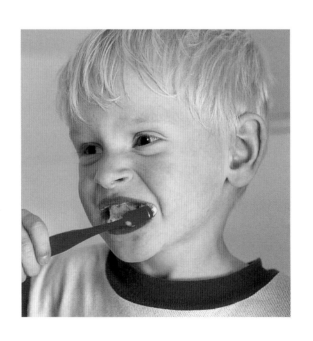

4

- Starting to clean

- Your growing child

- Get brushing right

- Choosing a toothbrush

Starting to clean

A healthy mouth is essential for your child's well-being, and a bright, confident smile will help her throughout her life. Dental care means more than just the teeth – caring for your child's gums is equally important, as these are the foundation for strong teeth. As well as regular visits to the dentist and a balanced diet, the best way to achieve a healthy mouth is by establishing a regular, thorough cleaning routine right from babyhood.

Your new baby

There is really no need to clean inside your new baby's mouth but you should adopt a regular oral hygiene routine using a small soft-headed toothbrush as soon as your child's first tooth erupts.

Cleaning the first teeth

As soon as your baby's first tooth emerges you need to clean it – and all the subsequent teeth – regularly twice a day, morning and at night after the final feed.

1 The best position in which to do this is to lie your baby on your lap so that you are looking down at her mouth from above.

2 Use a very thin film of toothpaste on a baby toothbrush and brush very gently but thoroughly all around the surfaces of the teeth and surrounding gums.

3 Always check the recommended age range on the toothbrush and toothpaste packet and use the brush with a light touch.

Your growing child

As your child grows you will find that she wants to be involved in the toothbrushing process herself, probably grabbing the toothbrush from you! This is fine and you should encourage any signs of enthusiasm, which will help establish toothbrushing as a regular habit.

It is important to remember that you still need to brush your child's teeth carefully yourself, as she won't have the necessary skills to do a thorough job herself.

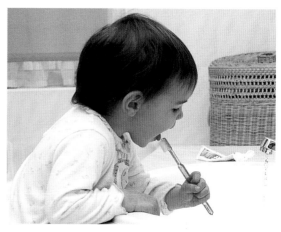

Brushing your toddler's teeth

1 Stand behind your toddler to brush her teeth, as this makes it easier for you to feel your way around her mouth with the brush.

2 You still need only a smear of toothpaste – certainly not enough to make any foam in your child's mouth. Any more than a pea-sized blob is too much, because toddlers do not yet have the co-ordination to manage spitting out the excess.

Above: A toddler will enjoy having a go himself, but you'll need to be on hand to ensure the job is done properly.

3 Encourage your child not to swallow the toothpaste, because too much fluoride could cause her developing permanent teeth to become discoloured (fluorosis). The aim is simply to bring the fluoride in the toothpaste into contact with your child's teeth which have already erupted to strengthen the enamel.

Brushing pre-schooler's teeth

1 For a pre-school child aged 3–5 years, stand behind him to brush his teeth. If he will let you, tilt his head backwards slightly to clean the top teeth, then ask him to look forwards while you brush the bottom teeth. Your child should be using a proper junior toothbrush by now, but you will still need to do the bulk of the brushing.

2 He will probably enjoy squeezing out his own toothpaste now, but it's essential to stick to pea-sized amounts for each brushing session as it is still easy for your child to accidentally swallow tooth-paste. You may find it easier to achieve this by using a pump-action toothpaste dispenser rather than a tube, in order to control the amount that comes out.

3 Your child is unlikely to be able to spit out toothpaste until he is 6 years old, but you can encourage him to do this by giving him a small cup so that he can get involved in rinsing his mouth.

Reluctant to brush?

From time to time, many toddlers and pre-schoolers will make toothbrushing a battleground. The tips below may help to smooth things along:
- Brush your own teeth at the same time as your child is brushing his.
- Pretend you can see the food in his mouth that needs to be brushed away and praise him when it's 'gone'.

- Put a mirror at your child's level so that he can watch himself brushing his teeth without you lifting him up. Alternatively, use a hand-held mirror.
- Let him choose his own novelty or favourite character toothbrush.
- Use a hand puppet as a 'friend' to brush his teeth with.
- Ask him to show you his 'tiger teeth', so that he snarls to reveal his front teeth ready for brushing.
- Always tell him how shiny his clean teeth look after brushing, and tell him what a good boy he is.

Below: Watching you brush your teeth is a sure-fire way of encouraging your baby to copy you!

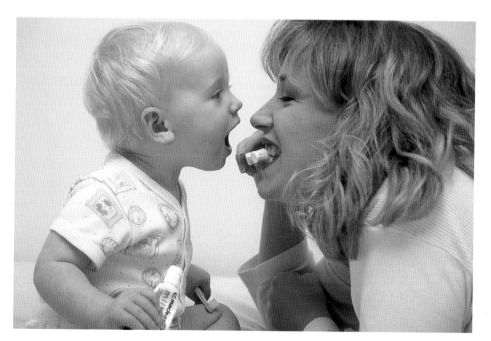

Get brushing right

Using the right technique when brushing your child's teeth can make a huge difference to how effective the routine is. The aim is to get rid of as much plaque as possible, without harming the teeth or gums in the process.

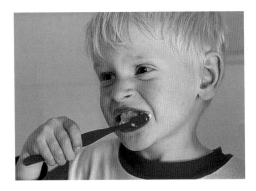

Above: If your child can see himself in a mirror he'll find it easier to get his brushing technique correct.

You need to exert even, gentle pressure when cleaning. Brushing too hard can wear away the tooth enamel over time, so encourage your child to take longer, but brush less firmly.

Cleaning all surfaces

There are three main surfaces to think about: the inside surfaces, the outside surfaces, and the flat chewing surfaces. Take special care to clean the back molars (tongue side) and the upper molars (cheek side), as these are the easiest for your child to miss when brushing.

Here is a step-by-step guide to help you get the brushing technique right:

1 Start with the outside surfaces of the top teeth, beginning at the back molars, then slowly move around to the centre and across to the other side. Hold the brush so that the bristles are at a slight angle to the gumline and move it in a gentle circular motion over one or two teeth at a time.

2 Next, clean the inside surfaces of the top teeth, working from the back to the centre and then around to the other side. Hold the brush vertically and use the front section of the brush, again with a gentle circular motion.

Keep watching

You will need to continue supervising your child's toothbrushing until he is at least 7 or 8 years old, and even then you may need to keep an eye on a child who is reluctant to do the job thoroughly.

3 Finally, brush the chewing surfaces, keeping the toothbrush flat so that you clean the grooves and natural fissures in the molars too.

4 Repeat for the teeth in the lower jaw.

Common questions

Q How can I show my child how to use a toothbrush?

A The best way is to ask your dentist to demonstrate in your child's own mouth, or at least ot show her using a set of demonstration teeth. But you can also help her to understand how much pressure to use by rubbing a toothbrush gently on the palm of her hand.

Q I never know when I've brushed my child's teeth enough. How can I tell?

A As long as you have brushed the surface of each tooth thoroughly, using a soft brush and fluoride toothpaste, it is likely that your child's teeth are fine. However, you may find it helpful to use some disclosing tablets to reveal remaining plaque. Your child should chew one (or a part of one) of these small pink or blue tablets for 30 seconds or so, then wash out her mouth with water and spit. The plaque on your child's teeth will then be stained pink or blue so that she can see where she needs to brush more carefully. These tablets are only suitable for children who can chew without swallowing and spit effectively. Always check the age-range on the box.

'My daughter is very unwilling to let me help her brush her teeth, but I have to replace her toothbrush very frequently as she manages to bite the bristles and makes them splay out sideways within a few days of having a new brush. I've insisted on "finishing off" her teeth when she's done her own brushing, but I can see it's going to take quite a while before she masters the right brushing technique on her own.'

Jane, mother of Maddie (4)

Choosing a toothbrush

What should you look for when choosing a toothbrush for your child? Nylon bristles are more hygienic than natural bristles and there are a number of other factors you need to consider.

The right toothbrush

- The bristles should be soft and the brushing head small so that it is easier for your child to reach all his teeth, including the very back ones.
- The brush should have a flat brushing surface, and look for rounded tips on the bristles so that they don't scratch the gums.
- Adult toothbrushes are not suitable for young children, as the brush head is too large to fit comfortably into a child's mouth and the bristles are likely to be too hard and abrasive.
- The type of toothbrush with a 'grippy' handle can help maximize motor skills.
- Keep the brushes upright in a place where they can dry out, and make sure they don't touch each other, as this can allow germs to pass from one brush to the other.
- Change your child's toothbrush when it shows signs of wear, such as the bristles splaying out.
- Get a new one every 4 months anyway, and certainly after an illness, as old brushes can harbour germs.

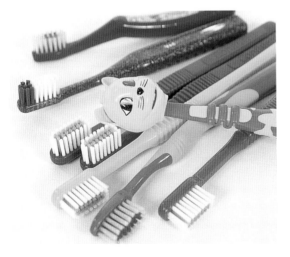

Left: A novelty toothbrush can be a great incentive for a child to brush properly.

Why toothpaste is important

A good toothpaste does several jobs at once:

1 Toothpaste is the cleaning agent that helps to remove particles of food from around the teeth and gums.

2 It usually contains fluoride, which helps to strengthen and protect the teeth from decay, and brushing brings fluoride into contact with the enamel surfaces of the teeth.

3 Using toothpaste leaves your child's mouth feeling fresh and clean.

For young children, you need to choose a toothpaste that is specially formulated for milk teeth. This will contain lower levels of fluoride than adult brands to avoid the risk of tooth discoloration (fluorosis). For extra reassurance, look for accreditation by a professional dental organization.

Too much fluoride?

Toothpaste is available in all sorts of flavours and attractive colours, which is great for encouraging a reluctant brusher. However, make sure your child understands that toothpaste shouldn't be swallowed, because ingesting too much fluoride may lead to fluorosis, a condition which can cause discoloration of the developing permanent teeth.

preventing decay

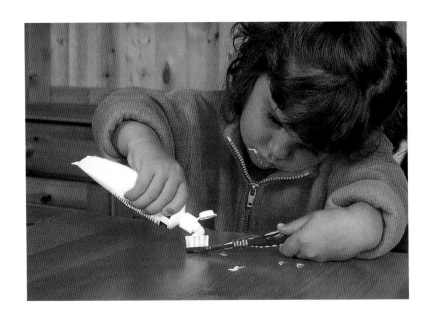

5

- Tooth decay explained

- Periodontal disease

- How to prevent tooth decay

Tooth decay explained

Dentists today put much more emphasis on preventive care than they used to in the past. This is because it has been proved that tooth decay, cavities and other problems are not inevitable at any age, and with the right cleaning routines and regular check-ups it is possible to keep teeth healthy and strong for a lifetime.

The cleansing power of saliva

Chewing produces saliva, which has a cleansing effect on your child's mouth. Offering crunchy snacks like celery or carrot encourages the production of saliva and barely increases the acid content of the mouth at all. Sugar-free gum is also an effective way of reducing the effect of the acid attack of food.

Many of the millions of germs in your mouth are perfectly harmless. The germs that are present in plaque and cause tooth decay love to eat sugar (especially refined sugar) and create acid as they do so. It is this acid that attacks the teeth.

What is decay?

Teeth have many natural resources to protect them from decay, but these defences can be broken down easily if the conditions are right.

Decay is caused by acids that eat into the surface of the tooth. Once the acid has broken through the enamel, the softer and more vulnerable inner part of the tooth (the dentine, see pages 25–26) is attacked, creating a hole in the tooth. Dentine is more easily dissolved than enamel, so once acid has reached it damage can be done very quickly. The cavity may be visible on the tooth's surface or it may be hidden between two teeth, which makes it unlikely that it will be spotted without an X-ray.

Eventually decay reaches the nerve of the tooth – and that's when it becomes painful. By this stage the tooth will definitely need treatment by your dentist because, once there is a hole, brushing alone is not enough to solve the problem. Decay in teeth can lead to infection, due to the breakdown products of the pulp once it has died as the result of tooth decay.

What causes it?

Plaque is the main culprit in tooth decay. This natural sticky substance forms continually on the teeth – run your tongue over your own teeth and you may feel a slightly rough film on the surface. This is plaque.

Plaque is made up of dead cells, tiny particles of food, bacteria, micro-organisms and a sticky part of saliva called mucin. You can remove it by careful brushing, but it is resistant to water so rinsing alone won't shift it. Plaque contains millions of bacteria, and when these come into contact with sucrose sugars in the mouth they start to form acids within seconds. It is these acids that attack the tooth enamel, and if left to get on with it they will eventually cause a hole to form.

If plaque is not removed it begins to calcify (harden) over a period of 2–12 days, forming a substance called calculus which builds up along the gumline. This is impossible to remove with a toothbrush and must be dealt with by a dentist or hygienist, who will use special scaling instruments to remove it.

The signs of decay

Here are the signs that could alert you to decay in your child's teeth or gums:

- Sensitivity to hot, cold and sweet things
- Pain which is spontaneous and may keep a child awake at night
- Stained pits and fissures
- A hole in a tooth

Periodontal disease

Gingivitis is the simplest form of periodontal disease and is even more common than tooth decay, but because it does not cause pain in the early stages it is often ignored by adults. It is caused by plaque collecting on the tooth. The gum responds by becoming red and swollen.

In the long term, periodontal disease can eventually result in the loss of teeth, as the bone and fibre structure holding them in place weakens and the teeth become loose. Some children – for example those with Down's syndrome – are more prone to periodontal disease and there are other rare conditions which result in premature destruction of the supporting structures of the teeth.

If you are already in the habit of brushing your child's gums as well as her teeth, she is unlikely to have problems with gum disease. The most obvious symptom is bleeding gums, and while this may seem alarming it can be cleared up by a couple of days of careful brushing. It is important to visit your dentist quickly if you suspect your child has gum disease.

Right: Gum disease is painful but it can be prevented by careful brushing twice a day.

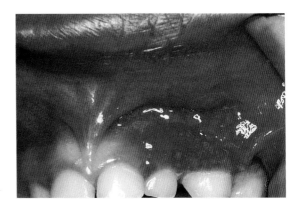

How to prevent decay

Prevention of decay depends on several factors. The two most important ones are regular brushing to avoid plaque accumulation and making sure you offer your child healthy food and drinks. You'll also need to make regular visits to the dentist a part of your family routine.

1 Brushing

The simplest way of helping to prevent decay is to establish a twice-daily brushing routine. The point of this is to remove plaque from the teeth.

When brushing, don't forget to brush close to the gumline to remove plaque from this area as well as from the surfaces of the teeth. Flossing is not appropriate for young children.

It is essential to brush your child's teeth last thing at night, and once this is done do not offer any further snacks or drinks other than water.

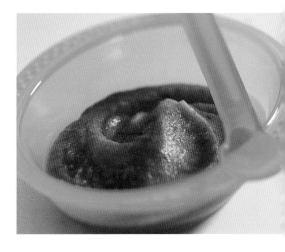

Above: *Puréeing simple vegetable and fruit meals is the best way to ensure your baby is getting a healthy diet right from the start.*

Sweet baby?

Take extra care when introducing your baby to solid foods – stick to savoury tastes to discourage an early sweet tooth. Check prepared baby food labels for sugar content. Better still, prepare and purée your own baby food so that you know exactly what has gone into it. Babies do not need any sugar (or salt) added to their food.

2 A good diet

What your child eats and drinks will have a significant effect on the health of his teeth. It is the sugars in food that help to form tooth-decaying acids. These are especially dangerous when they are sucrose sugars, like those found in processed foods, sweets and cakes. These are broken down more quickly in the mouth.

The key is to stick to three regular mealtimes to avoid snacks throughout the day. It is important to allow long periods between exposure to food to give the acids formed during eating time to become neutralized. This helps to reverse the demineralizing effects of acid on the tooth enamel. Regular family meals are often difficult to manage but do help to structure eating times.

In practice it is often hard for a toddler to go for long periods without food, and most health visitors would advise a number of healthy snacks throughout the day in order to meet your growing child's nutritional needs. So, if your child must eat between main meals, make sure you provide foods that won't ruin his teeth – for example, bread, breadsticks or cheese – and make sure he rinses his mouth afterwards with water.

Below: Encourage an older baby to enjoy healthy finger foods such as lightly cooked vegetable sticks and strips of toast.

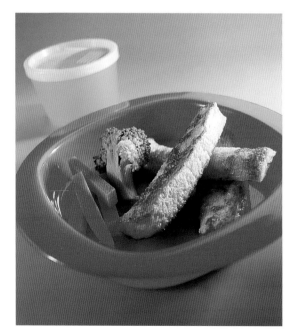

Sweets and treats

Sweets should be regarded as a once-a-week treat. Chocolate biscuits should be regarded as sweets too, and should be offered only on a once-a-week basis. Be aware of how much time your child's mouth spends bathed in sugary fluids. For example, if he sucks a packet of boiled sweets it is likely to be two hours or so before he's finished the pack, and his teeth will be coated in sugar throughout that time. A small bar of milk chocolate, on the other hand, is quickly eaten and the residues on his teeth will melt and be dissolved away by the saliva in his mouth. Make sure that your child cleans his teeth immediately afterwards.

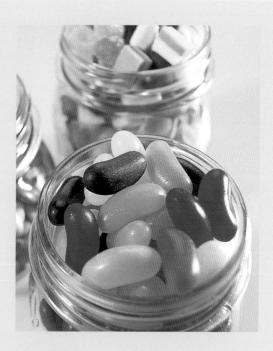

Above: Sweets attract all children, but you need to be vigilant about ensuring they're an occasional treat.

Hidden sugars

Becoming aware of how
much sugar is contained in
everyday foods will help
you to assess how much
and how often to give them.
Many foods contain sugar
that isn't labelled as clearly
as that: sucrose, maltose,
dextrose and fructose, for
example, are sugars by
another name. Also be
aware of hidden sugars in
medicines. Ask the
pharmacist to give you a
sugar-free version of
children's medicines
whenever they are
available as an option.

3 Watching drinks

What your child eats is not the only source of
harmful acids, which can also come from anything
she drinks other than water. Even milk contains
lactose, a natural sugar that forms acids if left in
contact with the teeth for too long – which is why it
is so important not to leave your baby or toddler
sucking on a breast or bottle when she goes to
sleep. There is a widely recognized form of decay
called 'rampant caries'
that is the direct result
of a baby spending
long periods sucking
on either a bottle or
the breast. To
protect your child's
teeth, you should

Right: Fruit juices
cause tooth erosion,
so try to stick to water
or milk instead.

aim to stop breast- and bottlefeeding at around 1 year old. For the same reason, never put anything sweet on a dummy to make it more tempting for your baby, as this will simply rot her teeth.

Fizzy drinks, squashes and fruit juices are all high in sugars and carbonic acids. Carbonated drinks and citric acid will cause erosion of the teeth. Ideally, fizzy drinks should be banned. Get your child into the water-drinking habit from babyhood.

Golden rules

- Do not introduce babies to juices.
- Encourage your child to use straws, as they direct the drink beyond the teeth and so help to protect them.
- Offer juices, preferably diluted, only at meal times. Orange juice increases iron absorption but is very acidic and may lead to tooth erosion.
- Encourage your child to avoid sweet drinks.
- If the use of fizzy drinks is unavoidable, then they should be saved for parties or special occasions rather than being given as a regular drink.

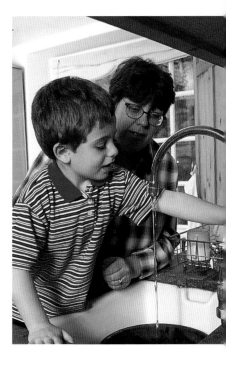

Above: Older children can begin to get drinks of water for themselves.

Drink up

Encourage your child to have a drink of fresh water after every meal or snack. This will help to clean food debris from between her teeth.

Move on up

Baby toothpastes may contain too little fluoride to offer enough protection for an older child's teeth, so always check the age range on the packaging and move up to adult toothpaste at around 8 years of age.

4 Fluoride

Fluoride may affect the teeth both during their development prior to their eruption and after they have emerged. Fluoride may have a local effect as it is absorbed by the surface of the teeth from toothpaste and mouthwash. It occurs naturally in the environment, but levels vary in different areas and water companies sometimes add extra fluoride to the water supply. Adding fluoride to tap water at an optimal level of 1ppm reduces dental decay by 50 per cent. Bottled mineral water often contains unspecified amounts of fluoride and other elements.

An obvious way to bring fluoride into contact with your child's teeth is to brush twice a day with a fluoride toothpaste. Remember to use a low-fluoride toothpaste for under-8s, as they could swallow it,

Sealants

When your child is approximately 6 years of age he will grow his first permanent molars. The chewing surfaces of these teeth are most vulnerable to decay. A popular and effective way to protect them is to seal the uneven biting surfaces (fissures) with a plastic sealant. This has to be done by your dentist but is an excellent way to prevent decay in the biting surface of the tooth, as plaque acid cannot penetrate the sealant. The new surface is also smoother and more even, making it easier to brush properly.

which may lead to a form of tooth discoloration called fluorosis in developing teeth.

As fluoride levels vary from one area to another, check local levels with your dentist, who can tell you if your child is getting sufficient supplies through water and toothpaste alone, or if a fluoride supplement might be advisable. You may also want to talk to the water company about the supply. Fluoride supplements are only recommended for at-risk children (i.e. at risk from decay because they have already suffered tooth decay, or at risk because of some overriding medical condition).

Below: A child only needs a smear of toothpaste, but she'll love squeezing the tube for herself – so you'll need to supervise!

5 Visiting the dentist

Get your baby used to visiting the dentist early on and continue to visit on a twice-yearly basis. This means that any problems or changes in your child's mouth can be identified and treated quickly, before they become serious. Familiarity also means that it is likely your child will not be afraid of dental visits as he gets older. A child-friendly dentist will have lots of simple ways to put your child at ease – for example, by offering stickers or 'polishing' his fingernails with the tooth-polishing equipment! For more details on finding a dentist, see pages 68–69.

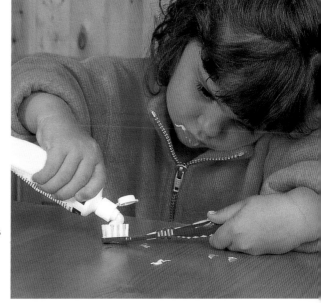

visiting the
dentist

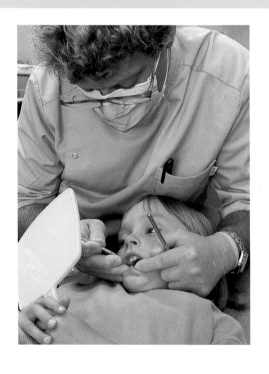

6

- Finding the right dentist

- The first visit

- First fillings

- Further visits and procedures

Finding the right dentist

Regular visits to the dentist are essential for your child's dental well-being. Whether you are already registered with a dentist or need to find a new one in your area, you can help your child by ensuring that her first visits to the dentist are confidence-building, happy experiences. Remember that prevention is always better than cure.

No matter how much care you take with your child's teeth, there may be times when you are faced with a problem. Always talk to your dentist or doctor if you have any worries about your child's teeth or general health.

What to look for

The right dentist is a child-friendly dentist – a person who feels comfortable being around children and knows how to put them at their ease in difficult circumstances. The best way to find one is through word-of-mouth recommendation. Alternatively, your doctor or health visitor may be able to suggest local dental practices, or you can look these up on the internet or in the telephone directory.

When you first make contact with the surgery, ask if the dentist is used to treating children. You may want to visit the surgery briefly before the appointment, so that you can let your child know what to expect. From the first appointment onwards, the dentist should be stressing prevention and good cleaning habits, and encouraging you and your child to adopt a sensible diet so that you can avoid any cavities right from the start.

Looking different

Remember to tell your child exactly what the dental examination room will look like. Mention the large chair, the overhead light, the sink to rinse in and the tray of dental instruments. It is also worth mentioning that the dentist will wear a mask over their mouth and nose, and rubber gloves on their hands.

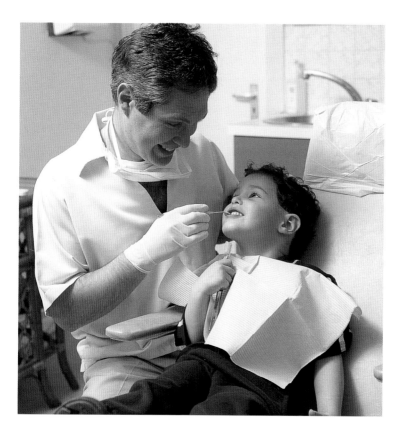

Left: *A child friendly dentist will help to make dental check-ups stress free.*

Information matters

When you register with a dentist you will be asked a number of questions about your child, including her medical history and when she last visited a dentist (if at all). It is essential to let your dentist know of any existing medical condition your child may have, any medication she takes regularly, and any operations she has had in the past. It is also important to mention any allergies, and whether your child has had any X-rays taken of her teeth in the past. All this information will help your dentist when deciding on appropriate treatment or any drugs that may need to be prescribed.

Waiting time

A good dentist should have a box of toys or books in the waiting room, but it is just as well to go supplied with some small toys, or books, or activities to distract your child in case you have to wait for a long time.

The first visit

You can take your baby along to the dentist as early as you like – ask the dentist at what age they first like to see children. However, it is likely that his first proper examination will be at around the age of 2.

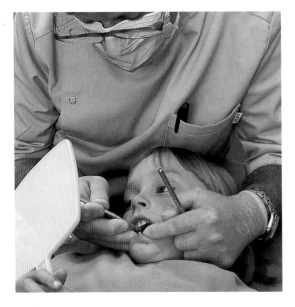

A good dentist will be calm and reassuring, and will try to make the visit a success by offering your child a 'ride' on the chair and a gentle polish (perhaps on his nails too). He may let him have a look in his own mouth with a mirror, and will present him with a sticker to take away.

It is important that your child feels relaxed, so the dentist should take time to let him look around and become familiar with the unfamiliar surroundings. They should also talk directly to him and explain clearly what is going to happen. Your child will

Above: Your dentist will examine your child's mouth to establish which teeth have already emerged.

Buzzy babies

Did you know that you can use an electric toothbrush even with a young toddler? In fact, it can be helpful to get him used to the feel of something buzzing inside his mouth, as this will make it far easier for the dentist to clean and polish his teeth later on.

Riding high
If your child is anxious about sitting in the dentist's chair, ask if he can sit on your lap for his first 'ride'. This will help him to feel secure as he will be experiencing a new sensation with you at hand.

need you to be there and you should also be made to feel welcome, but it is important that you let the dentist do the talking.

It is not possible for a dentist to examine, clean or treat your child's teeth unless your child is prepared to cooperate and feels confident. So, the dentist needs to build up a good relationship with your child right from the beginning. If the first time your child sees a dentist is when he has toothache caused by decay, he will inevitably be anxious, and this could set up a pattern of fear for the future.

What the dentist will do

On subsequent visits, the dentist will start by giving your child's teeth a thorough examination around every surface. A note will be made on his dental record of how many teeth have emerged and which have still to come through. The dentist will also check the health of your child's gums, which are a good indication of his overall dental health.

The dentist may offer you advice about cleaning your child's teeth and this is your opportunity to raise any concerns you may have, such as late teeth or wobbly teeth.

A polish will usually follow, with the dentist gently cleaning your child's teeth. If calculus (hardened plaque) has formed around his gum line, the dentist will remove this.

'I asked an experienced mum to recommend a child-friendly dentist. Before we went, we looked at a storybook about a visit to the dentist and I made sure they had seen me having a check-up too. Then I told them about the chair that goes up and down and all the bright lights they'd see. They ended up really looking forward to their first visit, and they loved the stickers the dentist gave them at the end.'

Sue, mother of Freddie (7) and Zoe (4)

First fillings

If, despite all your best efforts, your child does need a filling, don't get too upset about it and don't make her feel guilty. Talk to your dentist about the type of treatment your child will need and also about any changes you may need to make in her cleaning routine or diet. Your dentist should be very conscious of not frightening your child during any procedure, and this is where being familiar with the dental surgery from an early age comes into its own.

You will probably be informed about the problem during a regular check-up, or possibly through a dental check at your child's nursery, playgroup or school. You will be asked to make a separate appointment for the treatment, when your dentist will discuss with you in detail why the treatment is necessary, what to expect and the options for pain relief. In some cases, your dentist may refer your child to a paediatric dental specialist for treatment in a dedicated clinic or dental hospital.

Right: If there is a cavity, back teeth (or molars) are likely to be filled with a silver amalgam.

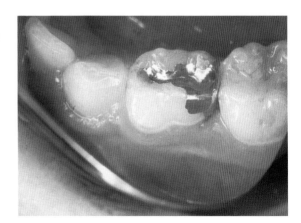

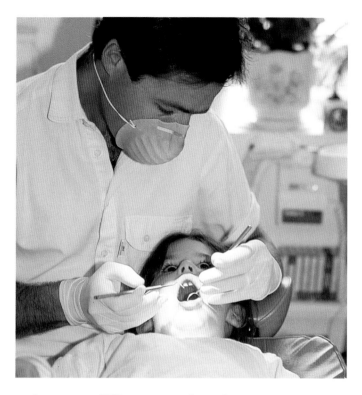

Left: Dentists need to protect both themselves and your child from infection, so they will wear a mask and gloves when giving treatment.

What are fillings made of?

There are several different types of filling from which your dentist can choose, though at present your child is most likely to be offered a silver amalgam filling for cavities in the back teeth (molars). Silver amalgam fillings have caused some controversy because, among other metals, they contain tiny amounts of mercury, which is poisonous. However, they are still considered safe and certainly last longer than other filling materials. On the more visible teeth, your dentist may use a white filling. These do not contain any metals but are not as long-lasting, although some have a fluoride-releasing function. Pre-formed stainless-steel crowns are a way of restoring a child's deciduous (baby) molars.

73

Further visits and procedures

Check-ups at the dentist are usually fairly speedy visits, but it may be that your child needs a longer session, or is given an appointment to come back at another time if extra treatment is needed. Occasionally you may be asked if you're willing for treatment to be given straight away, but you may prefer to have time to prepare your child.

General anaesthetics

In the rare cases where a general anaesthetic is needed for treatment – for example, for a difficult extraction where the child is unable to cooperate – this should be done in a hospital setting, where resuscitation facilities are to hand.

How often?

As long as you are brushing your child's teeth with a fluoride toothpaste twice a day, and eating a healthy diet, a check-up once every 6 months is usually enough for the dentist to keep track of your child's dental health and development. However, if there are specific problems or he has a cavity, more frequent visits will be required to carry out the treatment he needs.

Anaesthetics

If your child has a cavity that needs to be repaired, the dentist is likely to use a drill to remove any of the decay, leaving a clean hole which is then filled. This is likely to be uncomfortable, so a suitable local anaesthetic will be given before the treatment begins.

Local anaesthetic is injected into the gum to numb any sensation in the area that needs treatment. Your dentist may use a gel to numb the gum before giving this injection. The anaesthetic may take a little time to work, so you'll probably be asked to go back to the waiting room. The dentist should tell your child that his lips and tongue may feel strange, and that this sensation will last for a couple of hours, but that he'll be back to normal soon and must not chew the area while it feels 'funny'.

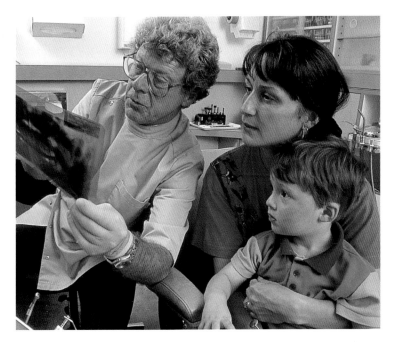

Left: The dentist will discuss your child's treatment with you and answer any questions you may have.

X-rays

If your child has an X-ray, this will reveal a lot of important information. It will not only show hidden areas of decay, but also the position and number of teeth that are still within the as well as the angle at which they will come through. It will also show any extra (or missing) teeth. All this information can give your dentist a good indication of whether future problems are likely or not.

With modern equipment the radiation dose is minimal, in many cases little more than sitting reasonably close to a colour television.

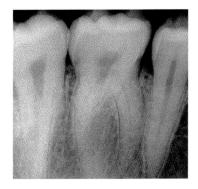

Above: An X-ray can reveal parts of your child's teeth that you wouldn't normally see!

other
problems
with teeth

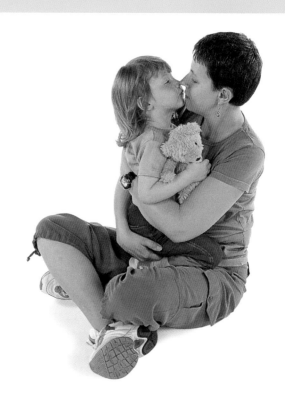

7

- Medical problems

- Other teeth troubles

- Losing or breaking a tooth

- Childhood habits

- When will they wobble?

- Problem-solving: questions and answers

Medical problems

Cavities are the most obvious problems that your dentist can resolve, but there are many other potential difficulties that can arise with a young child's teeth. Medical problems are first on the list. These include the following:

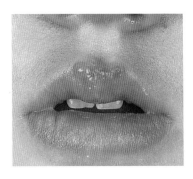

Above A cold sore can be uncomfortable and unsightly.

- **Heart problems.** Children with some types of heart disease have to be especially careful about dental hygiene. Infections can pass quickly from the gums into the blood stream, reaching the damaged heart. The dentist must be told about any pre-existing conditions, as it may be necessary to give antibiotics before beginning any dental treatment in order to protect the child from infection.
- **Diabetes.** Diabetes can mean a child takes longer to heal after any medical treatment, including dental work, so it is especially important to keep a diabetic child's teeth and gums scrupulously clean.
- **Down's syndrome.** Children with Down's syndrome may have a number of problems with their mouth, teeth and gums, including small teeth, missing teeth or disturbed enamel production, and a large tongue. A child with Down's needs to take especial care with cleaning and caring for the gums, and will need to be seen regularly for monitoring by the family dentist or a consultant. This is because Down's is also associated with heart problems, which can be directly affected by gum infections via the blood stream.
- **Cleft lip or palate.** During pregnancy, the two sides of the upper lip and roof of the baby's mouth fuse together. If this fails to happen there is a 'cleft' in the lip, the palate or both. You will be introduced to the cleft team, which will include a plastic craniofacial surgeon, an oral and maxillofacial surgeon, speech therapist, psychologist,

orthodontist and a paediatric dentist. Your child will need ongoing specialist care until she has stopped growing and reached adulthood.

- **Tongue tie.** In some babies, a membrane joins the tongue to the lower part of the mouth. Sometimes this results in your baby being unable to stick her tongue out properly. This is known as a 'tongue tie' and in rare cases may cause problems with speech and the removal of food from around the teeth. If you are concerned about this, speak to your doctor or health visitor.

- **Cold sores.** Cold sores are caused by the herpes virus and typically develop around the lips. They occur only if the child has previously experienced a 'primary herpetic gingivostomatitis' which presents as a feverish illness with painful mouth ulcers lasting 7–10 days. Cold sores may be treated by applying medication as soon as they begin. Speak to your dentist if this is a problem for your child.

- **Mouth ulcers.** These small lesions within the soft skin of the mouth and around the gums can be surprisingly painful. Using a dab of pain-relief gel can help, although you should read the dosage instructions carefully as there is a limit to how often you can use these safely. If mouth ulcers presents a big problem, see your dentist or doctor and ask for a referral to your local paediatric dentist.

- **Thrush.** White spots inside the mouth and on the tongue may indicate thrush, which may need antifungal treatment.

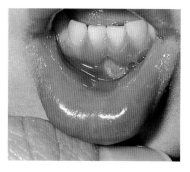

Above There are around 40 different types of mouth ulcers – if they are a recurring problem, talk to your dentist or doctor.

Medication update

Before starting any dental treatment, be sure to tell your dentist if your child is using any medication or has a medical problem.

Other teeth troubles

As your baby grows you may encounter other difficulties with her teeth that cause concern. Accidents may damage them, or poor feeding habits can eventually lead to decay. Other problems are caused by habits like tooth grinding that are difficult to break. Here are some of the key things to be aware of.

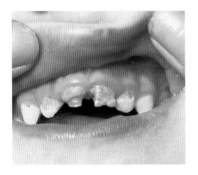

Above: *Constant sucking on a bottle of milk or juice can cause a type of decay known as 'bottle caries'.*

Baby bottle tooth decay

Once your baby can use a cup (from around 6–8 months old) don't give him drinks of milk or juice to sip at from a bottle, as this would leave his teeth coated with sticky or sugary fluids for long periods. This is especially important at night. Eventually this practice will cause decay, especially if you aren't already in a regular brushing and cleaning routine with your baby. Stick to water wherever possible.

It is important to remember that prolonged 'on-demand' breastfeeding can also lead to tooth decay in children older than 1 year.

Jaw relationship

Problems with jaw relationship may run in the family. However, your child's jaw could eventually become distorted by continued use of a dummy or bottle. Try to get rid of bottles and dummies after a year. Thumb or finger sucking may also cause a similar deformation of the upper jaw.

Overcrowding

Overcrowding is unlikely to be a problem with your child's milk teeth, but even if it is, it is unlikely that any treatment will be needed. Occasionally the first permanent molars become impacted into the second deciduous molars, in which case it may become necessary to see a paediatric dental specialist. Overcrowded milk teeth can be a predictor of future overcrowding problems with the permanent teeth, so your dentist will keep an eye on your child's progress.

Abscesses

An abscess is caused by the death of the pulp of a tooth. It is likely to be painful and may be accompanied by a fever and swelling of the affected area. In most cases the tooth will need to be removed. Your child will almost certainly be prescribed a course of antibiotics to clear the infection and it is important to finish the course, even if the pain is gone and the swelling has subsided.

Halitosis (bad breath)

If you are cleaning your child's teeth twice daily and he is eating a good, mixed diet, his breath shouldn't smell unpleasant. If it does and you are concerned, ask your dentist whether there is any obvious reason. If not, and the problem persists, you should see your doctor to rule out any medical causes.

Orthodontics

It is unlikely that your child will see an orthodontist before he has some permanent teeth. The earliest you might expect your child to have any orthodontic treatment is around 8 years old, when interceptive treatment may be offered.

Stained teeth

Permanent teeth may appear mottled if a child has ingested too much fluoride over a long period. Other stains or discoloration may be caused by tetracycline drugs taken by the mother during pregnancy or the child in the early years of life. This staining is an integral part of the structure of the tooth.

There is another form of stain that is caused – in part – by ineffective brushing and may be removed by your dentist.

If your child's teeth become stained, talk to your dentist about what is causing the problem. You may need professional help to get rid of the stains, but it is important to tackle them as your child can otherwise become very self-conscious about smiling.

'Dead' teeth

If your child's baby tooth is knocked and turns grey, there is no immediate need to take any action, and your dentist is unlikely to remove the tooth simply because it's discoloured. However, the tooth will need careful monitoring by your dentist as a dead tooth can become infected. This in turn could scar the permanent tooth that's not yet emerged. Your dentist will advise you what's best. If a permanent tooth becomes discoloured, it is also important to seek dental advice as soon as possible.

Losing a tooth

A milk tooth that is knocked out cannot be replanted – unlike a permanent tooth, which it may be possible to fix back into the jaw. You would normally be advised simply to wait for the permanent tooth to come through, but in exceptional cases a child may be fitted with dentures.

Delayed loss of baby teeth

Delayed loss of baby teeth, especially upper incisors, may occur as a result of previous trauma to the deciduous teeth, or because an extra (supernumerary) tooth is blocking the path of eruption of the permanent successor. X-ray examination is an important way of diagnosing the problem.

Chipped tooth

A chipped milk tooth may be built up using a composite resin but will need to be closely monitored because any damage to the tooth could leave it exposed to the risk of infection.

Tooth grinding

Some children grind their teeth in their sleep and there's not a great deal parents can do about this. However, if it's a serious problem the dentist may suggest your child wears a mouth guard at night – although it may not be possible to get your child to cooperate!

Wobbly teeth

If a tooth is loose enough your child will pull it out herself or, if she is willing, you can pull it out yourself. It is important to advise medical staff if your child has a wobbly tooth and is due to have a general anaesthetic.

'My daughter was referred to a paediatric dental hospital when she was 5. She needed a filling and they pursued a gently-gently approach, which involved lots of familiarization visits to build up her trust in the paediatric dentist before anything was done. She felt rather special on these visits and the filling went in without a murmur of protest.'

Sharon, mother of Frieda (5)

Losing or breaking a tooth

Any adult, let alone a parent, who has been around a young child for more than an hour or two will know just how active and lively they can be! Of course it's great for children to be on the go, but it's also essential to protect them as far as possible from obvious dangers.

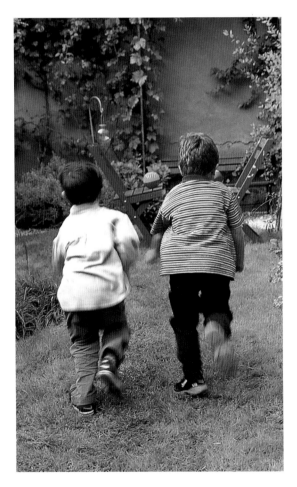

Young children are prone to accidents, and some of these can affect the teeth. Trips and falls can cause a tooth to be broken or knocked out, and damage to a milk tooth can potentially cause damage to the permanent tooth underneath it.

While it can be possible to reimplant a permanent tooth, this isn't possible with a milk tooth. However if your child breaks a portion of a tooth during a fall or accident, see your dentist as soon as possible as plastic bonding material may be able to be used to repair the damage. Of course it's best to avoid damage in the first place and, while you cannot have eyes in the back of your head, there are some obvious dangers you can avoid.

Left: *Check your garden carefully for any potential hazards – remember young children move very fast!*

Accident avoidance tactics

- Teach your child not to run around with anything in his mouth, such as a lolly stick, pen or toothbrush.
- Train him always to sit down when playing on a swing, and never to run in front of or behind a moving swing.
- If your toddler is learning to ride a tricycle, make sure it is stable and never let him ride it down a hill unattended.
- Be aware of stone steps, and always help your toddler up or down them.
- Encourage your child to run up hills, but not to run down them.

Right: *Always supervise a child who is learning to enjoy a new challenge, such as riding a tricycle.*

Childhood habits

Many children rely on comfort habits such as thumb or finger sucking or using a dummy, and these can eventually affect their teeth and jaw relationship. However, there is no need to stop your baby or toddler using these basic ways of comforting herself. The time to be concerned is if she is still spending hours sucking her thumb when she is ready to start school.

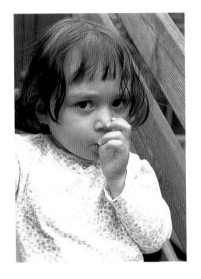

Above: Thumb-sucking is one of the most common childhood habits.

Even then, short periods are fine, but take common sense steps such as removing the thumb or dummy from your child's mouth once she is asleep. You will need to persuade her to drop the habit once her permanent teeth start coming through, as extended sucking will cause her teeth and jaw to become misaligned.

Other bad habits your child might slip into include lip, nail or cheek biting, or grinding her teeth. With any of these habits, you will have more success in persuading your child to drop it if you bring it to her attention in a matter-of-fact way each time you see her do it. Once she is conscious of what she is doing it may be easier to suggest that she stops. However, you may be in for the long haul in breaking some well-established habits.

Trying to stop?

If you are trying to persuade your child to drop a bad habit, ask your dentist to talk to her about it. A word of advice from a professional can be much more persuasive than nagging from you.

6 ways to cure a bad habit

Once your child has agreed that she would like to break a habit, these tips may help her on her way:

1 Use a gentle prompt. This might be a children's plaster over her thumb, which will remind her of what she is trying to achieve.

2 Make a star chart. Give one star for each successful day and offer a small treat at the end of every week.

3 Praise your child. Encouragement is always appreciated, so don't forget to tell her how pleased you are with all her efforts.

4 Tell your child how grown up she is being. Giving up a habit is difficult and she needs to know she's a 'big girl' for sticking at it.

5 Point out a potential role model. This might be an older cousin or the big sister of a friend, who has already given up a bad habit.

6 Consider a long-term incentive. For example, offer a special toy if she can stop her habit for a month.

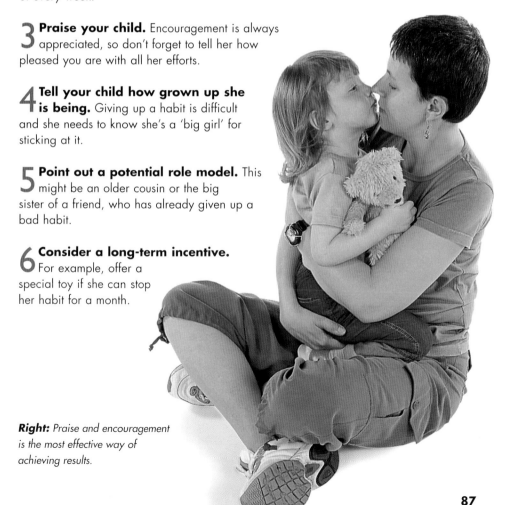

Right: Praise and encouragement is the most effective way of achieving results.

When will they wobble?

Sooner or later one of your child's milk teeth will begin to come loose as his permanent teeth start to emerge. This usually starts at around 6 years old, with the lower central incisors often being the first to go, followed by the upper central incisors.

Under anaesthetic

If your child needs a general anaesthetic in order to undergo an operation, check for a wobbly tooth in case he swallows it during the procedure.

The teeth on either side of the incisors will be the next to wobble, with the canines and molars last of all. Your child may be 11 or 12 years old (or even older), before all the primary teeth have gone.

If your child's wobbly tooth is interfering with his ability to eat or clean his teeth comfortably, you can help it along by pulling it out yourself, with two clean fingers. If you don't want to do this, ask your dentist for help. Most children are willing enough, with the promise of a visit from the tooth fairy to come.

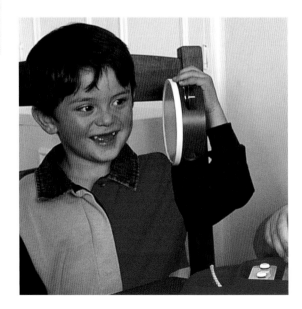

Right: A wobbly tooth is usually something your child will be very proud of – don't forget to take a few pictures of those endearing gaps!

Problem-solving:
questions and answers

Q My child has a lisp and while this isn't a worry at the moment, I'm afraid he'll be teased when he starts school. Is there anything I can do to help?

A Most toddlers don't form their words properly to begin with, but if you feel your child has a real problem, talk to your dentist to see if there are any obvious cause. However, speech difficulties are usually best dealt with by help from a speech therapist, who can give your child specific exercises to encourage him to form the right muscular movements as he speaks.

Q My 7-month-old baby won't settle without a dummy. Could this damage his milk teeth?

A Sucking comes very naturally to babies and it is quite normal for your baby to be soothed by feeding or sucking on a dummy. At this stage you don't need to worry about his teeth, but try to limit use of the dummy to bed and nap times. Once he's asleep, gently remove the dummy from his mouth. You should be aiming to part company with bottles and dummies soon after your baby is 1 year old, although this is often easier said than done. Try introducing a beaker now, and never sweeten the dummy before giving it to your child, as this will inevitably cause decay. Also bear in mind that your baby can't make vocal sounds when he is sucking a dummy, and this could discourage him from the pre-talking babble that is so important for early speech development. This becomes even more of an issue with an older baby.

Q I don't like the idea of giving my baby any unnecessary medication, but is it worth trying a homoeopathic remedy for teething?

A Teething gels and infant paracetamol are normally the only medications you would think about giving a teething baby, and both of these are considered safe. However, you can certainly try a homoeopathic remedy, such as teething granules. Make sure you buy these from a reputable homoeopath or pharmacy, and always read the instructions carefully before offering them to your baby.

Q Why does my baby dribble so much?

A A baby does not yet have sufficient muscular control in her mouth to allow her to swallow excess saliva, as an adult would. So, if she's making lots of extra saliva during teething there is nowhere for it to go but out and down her chin! You may want to use a soft, plastic-backed bib to catch the dribbles and keep her dry. A smear of petroleum jelly is also helpful to prevent her chin becoming sore.

Q My 9-month-old baby doesn't seem to like lumpy food. Is it OK to carry on giving her purées?

A Nutritionally your baby will be doing fine on puréed meals, but by this age it is important for her to start developing her chewing technique, even if she doesn't yet have any teeth. Her gums are hard enough to chew lumpy foods. The best way to encourage your baby's interest in taking more textured foods is to offer her finger foods she can hold herself, such as toast strips, pieces of cheese, thinly sliced apple and pear, and grated carrot.

Q I was always afraid of the dentist as a child but I don't want to pass on my fears to my own children. What should I do?

A If you are aware that your child is picking up on your own anxieties about the dentist, it may be best to ask your partner or a grandparent to accompany her for the first few visits. Find a dentist who specializes in working with young children and will take time and trouble over putting your child at her ease before beginning any examination or treatment. In the meantime, don't neglect your own dental health. Make an appointment for yourself separately and tell the dentist about your anxieties.

If you can be relaxed during your own dental treatment, let your child get used to the clinical surroundings of the dentist's surgery by taking her along on your own visits while she is a baby. Make sure she is safe and secure in her pushchair or car seat while you have your treatment.

Right: Your baby will pick up on your feelings, so try to stay positive even if you are scared of the dentist yourself.

Top 10 tips

A lifetime of healthy teeth and gums is a wonderful gift to give your child, and by following all the advice in this book, you'll be well on the way to making it happen. Remember these key things:

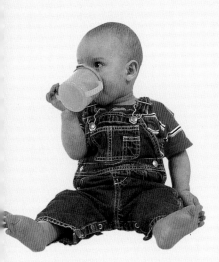

1 Start brushing your baby's teeth as soon as they appear. Use a soft-bristled brush and a toothpaste that's formulated for milk teeth.

2 Brush your child's teeth and gums regularly twice a day with a fluoride toothpaste to avoid a build-up of plaque.

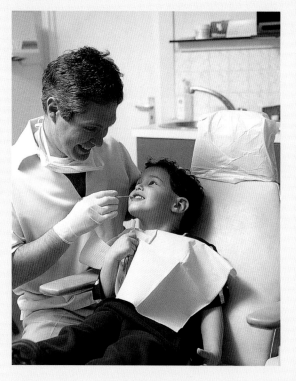

3 Stop giving bottles after the age of one year – use a beaker instead. Bottle or breastfeeding after 12 months can start to cause tooth decay.

4 Visit your dentist twice a year for check-ups. Getting your child used to these regular visits will establish good habits for future years.

5 Offer your child healthy meals, with plenty of fresh fruit and vegetables. Check food labels carefully to avoid hidden sugars.

6 Keep sweets and chocolate biscuits as a once-a-week treat. They bathe your child's teeth in the sticky sugars that quickly build up acids which will attack the tooth enamel.

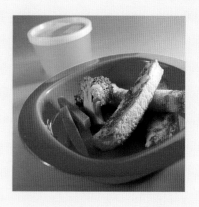

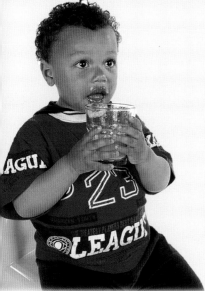

7 Stick to water or milk as your child's regular drinks.

8 Try to keep to regular mealtimes rather than all-day snacking. This means your child will not have food continually in contact with her teeth.

9 Take basic safety precautions at home and in the garden to avoid accidents. A milk tooth that falls out cannot be reimplanted.

10 Set your child a good example by letting her see you taking care over your own dental hygiene. Brushing your teeth together is a great way to encourage a reluctant toddler to get involved.

Index

a

abscesses 29, 81
accidents 84
    avoiding 85, 93
alcohol consumption in pregnancy
    14
allergies 19, 69
antibiotics 12, 78, 81

b

babies
    brushing teeth 46, 92
    development 10, 11, 29
    dribbling 90
    preventing tooth decay 59, 92
    see also bottlefeeding;
        breastfeeding; teething
bad breath (halitosis) 81
bottlefeeding 32–3, 62–3, 80,
    92
breastfeeding 11, 30–1, 32, 42
    and tooth decay 62–3, 80, 92
brushing teeth 6, 44–53, 92
    babies 46, 92
    and gums 27
    pre-schoolers 48
    in pregnancy 18
    reluctance to brush 48–9
    technique 50–1
    toddlers 47, 70, 93
    toothbrushes 52, 70
    toothpaste 53, 64, 64–5

c

chipped teeth 83
cleft lip or palate 78–9
cold sores 79
colour of teeth 25

d

decay see tooth decay
dental treatment 6–7, 66–75
    anaesthetics 71, 88

check-ups 71, 74, 92
child-friendly dentists 65, 68, 69,
    71
fear of dentists 91
fillings 12, 72–3
first visits 70–1
giving information to the dentist
    69
in pregnancy 10, 11, 12, 15
telling children what to expect 68,
    71
waiting time 69
X-rays 75
diabetes 78
diet see food
Down's syndrome children 58, 78
drinks 41, 62–3, 93
drugs see medicines
dummies 27, 41, 63, 80
    breaking the habit 86, 89

e

electric toothbrushes 70
exercise in pregnancy 14

f

fatty acids 15
feeding
    and teething 39
    and tooth development 29,
        30–3
    see also bottlefeeding;
        breastfeeding
fillings 72–3
fluoride 64–5, 92
fluorosis 47, 53, 64
folic acid 14
food
    babies and lumpy foods 90
    in pregnancy
        food hygiene and preparation
            18–19
        healthy eating 14–17

sweets and sugary foods 59, 60, 62, 93
and teething 36, 43

g
general anaesthetics 71, 88
gum disease 58
gums 27

h
habits, curing a bad habit 86–7
halitosis (bad breath) 81
healthy eating *see* food
heart problems 78
homoeopathic remedies 90
hospitals 74, 83

j
jaw development 11, 27
jaw relationship 80

m
medical problems 78–9
medicines
    antibiotics 12, 78, 81
    hidden sugars in 62
    homoeopathic 90
    infant paracetamol 39, 43, 90
    and tooth development 12
mercury, and dental fillings 12
milk teeth
    accidents and breakages 84–5, 93
    chipped 83
    `dead' 82
    delayed loss of 83
    first tooth 6, 7, 32
    infections and abscesses 29, 91
    losing 23, 82–3
    maintaining spacing 28
    order of emergence 22, 23, 24
    overcrowded 80–1
    wobbly 83, 88

see also brushing teeth
mouth ulcers 79

n
newborn (natal) teeth 13

o
orthodontics 81

p
pain, relieving teething pain 42–3
permanent teeth 29, 64, 82
    and fluorosis 47, 53
plaque 27, 57
    disclosing tablets 51
pregnancy 6, 8–19
    care of the teeth in 18
    dental treatment in 10, 12, 15
    and diet 14–19
    infections in 12
    and tooth development 10, 12–13
premature birth 12

q
questions and answers 89–91

r
root formation 10

s
saliva 33, 56
sealants 64
sleeping, and teething 41
smoking in pregnancy 14
speech problems 89
spina bifida 14
stained teeth 82
sucking reflex 11

t
teething 34–43
    crooked teeth 39
    and dummies 41

relieving pain 42–3
seeing the new tooth 37
signs of 36–7
soothing your baby 40–1
teething rings 42
thrush 79
thumb-sucking 7, 11, 80, 86, 87
toddlers 6
avoiding accidents 84, 85
cleaning teeth 47, 70, 93
speech problems 89
tongue tie 79
tooth decay 54–65
bottle caries 32, 80
causes of 57
defining 56
periodontal disease 58
preventing 59–65, 92, 93
signs of 57
tooth development 10, 20–33
canines 22, 24, 88

cementum 25, 26
central incisors 22, 24, 88
dentine 25–6, 56
enamel 10, 25
factors affecting 12–13
and feeding 29, 30–3
lateral incisors 22, 24
molars 22, 24, 64, 88
periodontal ligament 25
pulp 25, 26
supporting fibres 25, 26
see also milk teeth
toothbrushes 52, 70
toothpaste 52, 64–5, 92
toys, chewing 36

W

wobbly teeth 83, 88

X

X-rays 13, 75

Acknowledgements

Bubbles 69, 92 right, /Clarissa
Leahy 73, /Daniel Pangbourne 8,
/Claire Paxton 27, /Toni Revan 1,
47, /Loisjoy Thurston 7, /Ian West
44, 50.
Getty Images/Elizabeth Young 40.
**Octopus Publishing Group
Limited**/David Jordan 59, 60, 61,
/Peter Pugh-Cook 2, 5, 11, 20, 23,
28, 29, 31, 33, 35, 36, 37, 38,
42, 52, 54, 62, 63, 65, 76, 84,
85, 86, 87, 88, 91, 92 centre left,
93 top right, 93 bottom left,
/William Reavell 19.
Angela Hampton/Family Life Picture
Library 49.
Photodisc 15.
© **Dr B.Scheer** 72.

Science Photo Library/St
Bartholomew's Hospital 78, /Scott
Camazine 13, /Dr P.Marazzi 79
/Vanessa Vick 75 bottom, /Hattie
Young 66, 70, 75 top, The
Wellcome Photo Library 58, 80.

Executive Editor Jane McIntosh
Excutive Art Editor Joanna Bennett
Designer Bill Mason
Production Controller Viv Cracknell
Picture Librarian Zoë Holtermann
Photography Peter Pugh-Cook